Diabetic Smoothie Recipes

35 Easy & Delicious Smoothie Recipes for Diabetics

TABLE of CONTENTS

Introduction

I would like to thank you for purchasing this book, 'Diabetic Smoothie Recipes - 35 Easy & Delicious Smoothie Recipes for Diabetics.'

This book is your guide to leading a healthy and happy life as a diabetic. Diabetes is a long-term metabolic disorder that causes an individual to have high blood sugar (glucose) due to either of two reasons - Insulin isn't being produced adequately or the cells in the body are not properly responding to insulin or both.

Diabetes causes rather uncomfortable symptoms like frequent urination, acute hunger, and thirst, weight loss that is unusual and tingling in the hands and feet. There are usually 2 types of diabetes - Type 1 in which the body fails to produce insulin and Type 2 in which the body doesn't produce enough insulin. Gestational diabetes is a type of diabetes that occurs in pregnant women and can cause pregnancy complications.

Keeping blood sugar under control is the major concern for a diabetic. It is a chronic illness, but managing it can be made easier by monitoring your diet. Having diabetes doesn't mean you that have to sacrifice all your favorite foods though. There is always a healthier substitute that you can use so that you can avoid the unnecessary sugar spike.

Consuming hearty, well-balanced meals can assist in maintaining a steady level of blood sugar. A nutritionist or dietitian can guide you with a wholesome plan that will include a lot of super foods like green leafy vegetables, whole grains, berries, citrus, dairies like Greek yogurt and almond milk, nuts and natural nut butter.

The best way to integrate all these nutritious foods into your diet is turning it into a delicious smoothie. You can have a smoothie every day because it is very filling and you can have it on the go. Just make sure you count the fruits that you put into the smoothie as part of your allowance so that you don't go overboard. Smoothies are quick and easy to make. You just have to throw everything in the blender and you get a glass of pure goodness, which is appetizing as well as delicious.

Smoothies are a great way to control your cravings and satisfy your sweet tooth. It makes you feel energetic all day and improves mental clarity, concentration, focus and memory. These healthy drinks contain berries that are rich in antioxidants and avocados and leafy greens, which have healthy fats.

The recipes for smoothies mentioned in this book will make sure that your body gets all the necessary vitamins, minerals, fibers and antioxidants that it needs and keep your blood sugar level low while slowing down the absorption of glucose and detoxify the body. There are a variety of smoothies out there but this book is just for all the diabetics who are fed up with their restricted diets. These recipes are not only easy but are quite delicious as well. You just need to stock up your pantry with the necessary ingredients. The ingredients used are also easily available in your local super market, so you don't have to worry about having to use some exotic fruits or other such ingredients. For best results, use fresh and organic ingredients. To make it easy on your pocket, you can buy these fruits in bulk and freeze them and use them accordingly. That's it – that is all you need to get the best from your smoothies.

So, get ready to tickle your taste buds and have a fulfilling beginning, mid-day snack or dessert for the day with these delectable smoothies that can be whipped up from easily available ingredients in the market and are light on your pocket as well as beneficial for your metabolism.

Let the recipes in this book lead the way towards a happier and a healthier life!

<u>Pro-tip</u>: Preferably use natural sweeteners like Stevia for sweetening the smoothies. Avoid using fruits that have more sugar content in it.

KALE AND CUCUMBER SALAD SMOOTHIE

Serves: 2

Ingredients:

- 2 stalks kale
- 6 baby carrots
- 1 small onion
- A handful parsley
- 1 apple
- 2 cups water
- 1 small cucumber
- 2 medium tomatoes
- 1 ripe avocado
- 2 tablespoons lemon juice

Method:

1. Discard hard stems and ribs of kale. Tear the leaves. Rinse and chop the baby carrots.
2. Peel and quarter the onion. Rinse parsley. Peel and core the apple. Chop apple into pieces.
3. Chop cucumber and tomatoes. Peel the avocado. Pit the avocado and chop into pieces.
4. Add kale, carrots, onion, parsley, apple, water, and cucumber, tomatoes, avocado and lemon juice into a

blender.

5. Blend for 30-40 seconds or until smooth. Add more water if you desire a smoothie of thinner consistency.

6. Pour into tall glasses and garnish with slices of cucumber or avocado.

7. Serve with crushed ice.

Rock melon Soya and Flax Smoothie

Serves: 2

Ingredients:

- 1 cup rock melon + extra to garnish
- 1 tablespoon flaxseeds
- 1 cup soy milk
- ½ cup crushed ice

Method:

1. Peel and deseed the rock melon. Chop into pieces.
2. Add rock melon, flaxseeds, and soy milk into a blender.
3. Blend for 30-40 seconds or until smooth. Add more soy milk if you desire a smoothie of thinner consistency.
4. Pour into tall glasses and garnish with slices of rock melon.
5. Serve with crushed ice.

<u>SUPERFOOD SMOOTHIE</u>

Serves: 2

Ingredients:

- 1 ½ cups almond milk, unsweetened
- 2/3 cup strawberries
- 1 cup blueberries
- 1 ripe avocado
- 1 cup spinach
- 1 cup berry yogurt
- 2 tablespoons chia seeds
- 2 teaspoons flaxseeds
- 2 scoops greens superfood
- 2 scoops diabetic friendly protein powder
- Ice cubes as required

Method:

1. Peel and pit the avocado. Chop into pieces.
2. Tear the spinach leaves.
3. Add almond milk, strawberries, blueberries, avocado, spinach, berry yogurt, chia seeds, flaxseeds, greens superfood, protein powder and ice cubes into a blender.
4. Blend for 30-40 seconds or until smooth. Add more almond milk if you desire a smoothie of thinner consistency.
5. Pour into tall glasses and garnish with slices of avocado.

Low Sugar Strawberry Smoothie

Serves: 2

Ingredients:

- 2 cups spinach
- 10 strawberries
- 2/3 cup cooked oats
- ½ cup plain Greek yogurt
- 2 tablespoons chia seeds
- 2 cups soy milk
- Stevia to taste
- Crushed ice

Method:

1. Rinse spinach and strawberries. Chop the spinach. Hull and slice the strawberries. Retain 2 slices strawberries to garnish.
2. Add all the ingredients into a blender. Blend for 30-40 seconds or until smooth. Add more soy milk if you desire a smoothie of thinner consistency.
3. Pour into tall glasses. Garnish with slices of strawberry and serve with crushed ice.

Peach Smoothie

Serves: 1

Ingredients:

- 1 small fresh or frozen peach
- ¼ teaspoon ground cinnamon
- 1 cup non-fat vanilla yogurt
- ¼ cup skim milk
- ½ cup ice cubes
- 1 slice strawberry

Method:

1. If you are using fresh peach, peel and deseed it. Chop into pieces.
2. Add peach, cinnamon, vanilla yogurt, skim milk and ice cubes into a blender.
3. Blend for 30-40 seconds or until smooth.
4. Pour into a tall glass and garnish with a slice of strawberry.

Bloody Mary Smoothie

Serves: 2

Ingredients:

- 1 large tomato
- 2 cups of tomato juice
- 1 medium sized cucumber
- Juice of a lemon
- 1 teaspoon Sriracha sauce
- 3 teaspoons Worcestershire sauce
- 2 thin slices lemon

Method:

1. Peel and chop the cucumber. Chop the tomato.
2. Add tomato, tomato juice, cucumber, lemon juice, sriracha sauce and Worcestershire sauce into a blender. Blend for 30-40 seconds or until smooth.
3. Pour into tall glasses garnished with thin slices of lemon and serve with crushed ice.

<u>**SNICKERS SMOOTHIE**</u>

Serves: 2

Ingredients:

- 1 cup plain yogurt, unsweetened or plain kefir, unsweetened
- 2 cups almond milk, unsweetened
- Stevia to taste
- 10 drops English toffee Stevia
- 2 tablespoons cocoa powder, unsweetened
- 2 heaping tablespoons peanut butter or almond butter, unsweetened
- 2 tablespoons diabetic friendly vanilla protein powder
- 2 tablespoons chia seeds or ground flaxseed meal
- 1 teaspoon vanilla extract
- Ice cubes as required
- Roasted peanuts, crushed to garnish

Method:

1. Add yogurt, almond milk, Stevia, English toffee Stevia, cocoa powder, peanut butter, vanilla protein powder, chia seeds, vanilla extract and ice cubes into a blender.
2. Blend for 30-40 seconds or until smooth.
3. Pour into tall glasses and garnish with roasted crushed peanuts.

Diabetic Green Smoothie

Serves: 2

Ingredients:

- ½ cup fresh mint
- ½ cup flat leaf parsley
- 2 cups kale
- 1 large pear
- 1 stalk celery
- 1 medium cucumber
- 2 cups coconut water
- Cucumber slices to garnish

Method:

1. Remove the hard ribs and stems of kale. Chop the kale.
2. Peel the pear and chop into pieces. Chop cucumber into pieces. Rinse mint and parsley. Chop celery into pieces.
3. Add mint, parsley, kale, pear, celery, and cucumber and coconut water into a blender. Blend for 30-40 seconds or until smooth. Add more coconut water if you desire a smoothie of thinner consistency.
4. You can replace coconut water with yogurt or any milk of your choice.
5. Pour into tall glasses and garnish with cucumber slices.
6. Serve with crushed ice.

STRAWBERRY BANANA FLAXSEED SMOOTHIE

Serves: 1

Ingredients:

- ¾ cup fresh strawberries
- ¼ cup soft tofu
- 1 tablespoon skim milk
- ½ small banana
- 1 tablespoon ground flaxseeds
- 1 teaspoon honey
- ½ cup ice cubes

Method:

1. Hull and chop the strawberries. Peel and slice the banana.
2. Add strawberries, tofu, skim milk, banana, flaxseeds, honey and ice cubes into a blender.
3. Blend for 30-40 seconds or until smooth. Add more skim milk if you want a smoothie of thinner consistency.
4. Pour into a tall glass and serve.

Cherry Berry Oatmeal Smoothie

Serves: 2

Ingredients:

- 4 tablespoons quick cooking rolled oats
- 1/3 cup water
- 1/3 cup almond milk or skim milk
- 2 tablespoons almond butter
- 2 teaspoons honey
- ½ cup cherries, fresh or frozen
- ½ cup fresh or frozen strawberries
- Ice cubes as required

Method:

1. If you are using fresh strawberries, hull and chop into pieces. If you are using frozen, then partially thaw it.
2. If you are using fresh cherries, pit the cherries. If you are using frozen, then partially thaw it.
3. Add water and oats into a microwave safe bowl. Microwave on high for 40-60 seconds or until cooked. Remove from the microwave and cool completely.
4. Add the cooked oats, strawberries, cherries, almond milk, almond butter and honey.
4. Blend for 30-40 seconds or until smooth. Add ice cubes and blend again.
5. Pour into tall glasses and garnish with strawberry slices.

Easy Nectarine, Mixed Berry and Coconut Shake

Serves: 2

Ingredients:

- ¼ cup strawberries
- ¼ cup blueberries
- ¼ cup raspberries
- ¼ cup blackberries
- 2 medium nectarines
- 1 cup coconut water

Method:

1. Peel and deseed the nectarines. Chop the nectarines into pieces.
2. Add coconut water, strawberries, blueberries, raspberries, black berries and nectarines into a blender. Blend for 30-40 seconds or until smooth. Add more coconut water if you like a smoothie of thinner consistency.
3. Pour into tall glasses and serve with crushed ice.

DIABETIC OATMEAL BREAKFAST SMOOTHIE

Serves: 1

Ingredients:

- ½ cup uncooked oats
- 1 ½ cups skim milk
- 1 banana
- 1 tablespoon ground flaxseed
- 1 teaspoon coffee extract
- Stevia or Splenda to taste

Method:

1. Grind the oats in a spice grinder or coffee grinder.
2. Peel and slice the bananas. Freeze the banana slices.
3. Add ground oats, banana, skim milk, flaxseed, Stevia and coffee extract into a blender.
4. Blend for 30-40 seconds or until smooth. Add more skim milk if you like a smoothie of thinner consistency.
5. Pour into tall glasses and serve with crushed ice.

Berries and Almond Smoothie

Serves: 2

Ingredients:

- ¼ cup strawberries
- ¼ cup blueberries
- ¼ cup raspberries
- ¼ cup blackberries
- 4 medium fennel bulbs
- 2 tablespoons sunflower seeds
- 1 cup almond milk

Method:

1. Shred the fennel bulbs.
2. Add strawberries, blueberries, raspberries, black berries, fennel bulb, sunflower seeds and almond milk into a blender. Blend for 30-40 seconds or until smooth. Add more almond milk   if you like a smoothie of thinner consistency.
3. Pour into tall glasses and serve with crushed ice.

<u>**GREENIE GREEN SMOOTHIE**</u>

Serves: 2

Ingredients:

- 2 cups water
- 1 large ripe green pear
- 1 large ripe green apple
- A handful fresh mint
- 1 cup fresh kale or spinach
- 15 chilled green or moscato grapes
- Stevia to taste or truvia to taste
- 2-3 tablespoons lime juice
- 1 teaspoon ground cinnamon
- Ice cubes as required

Method:

1. Remove the hard ribs and stems of kale. Chop the kale.
2. Peel the pear and chop into pieces. Rinse mint and chop.
3. Core and chop the apple into pieces.
4. Add mint, kale, pear, water apple, grapes, Stevia, lime juice and cinnamon into a blender. Blend for 30-40 seconds or until smooth.
5. Add ice and blend again. Add more water if you desire a smoothie of thinner consistency.
6. Pour into tall glasses. Sprinkle some cinnamon on top.
7. Garnish with thin apple slices and serve.

Don't forget to like this book and leave a review!

Kiwi Fruit, Lemon, Lettuce and Green Tea Smoothie

Serves: 2

Ingredients:

- 2 medium kiwi fruits
- 6 lettuce leaves
- 1 ½ cups freshly brewed green tea
- ¼ cup lemon juice

Method:

1. Peel and chop the kiwi fruits. Rinse and tear the lettuce leaves.
2. Add kiwi fruits, lettuce leaves, green tea and lemon juice into a blender. Blend for about 20-30 seconds or until smooth.
3. Pour into tall glasses and serve with crushed ice.

Peanut Butter and Blueberry Smoothie

Serves: 1

Ingredients:

- 3 ounces light soft silken tofu
- 1 ¼ cups vanilla almond milk, unsweetened, chilled
- 1/3 cup frozen blueberries
- 8-10 grapes, chilled
- 1 tablespoon peanut butter
- Fresh blueberries to garnish
- Ice cubes as required

Method:

1. Add tofu, almond milk, frozen blueberries, grapes and peanut butter into a blender.
2. Blend for 30-40 seconds until smooth. Add ice cubes and blend again.
3. Pour into a tall glass. Garnish with fresh blueberries and serve.

Orange Dream Creamsicle

Serves: 2

Ingredients:

- 2 oranges
- ½ cup frozen orange juice
- ½ cup fat free yogurt
- ½ teaspoon vanilla extract
- Crushed ice

Method:

1. Peel and deseed the oranges. Chop the oranges into pieces.
2. Add orange, orange juice, yogurt, and vanilla extract into a blender. Blend for 30-40 seconds or until smooth. Add more orange juice if you like a smoothie of thinner consistency.
3. Pour into tall glasses and serve with crushed ice.

Blushing Julius

Serves: 2

Ingredients:

- 6 ounces soft silken tofu
- 1/3 cup non-fat dry milk powder
- 2 teaspoons honey
- 1 cup fresh orange juice, chilled
- 4 frozen strawberries
- ½ teaspoon vanilla extract
- Ice cubes as required
- Fresh strawberry slices to garnish

Method:

1. Add tofu, milk powder, honey, orange juice, strawberries and vanilla extract into a blender.
2. Blend for 30-40 seconds until smooth. Add ice cubes and blend again.
3. Pour into tall glasses. Garnish with fresh strawberry slices and serve.

BERRIES AND TOFU SHAKE

Serves: 2

Ingredients:

- ½ cup silken tofu
- ½ cup acai berries
- 1 cup soy milk
- 1 cup water
- 1 cup strawberries

Method:

1. Hull and slice chop the strawberries.
2. Add tofu, acai berries, soy milk, water and strawberries into a blender. Blend for 30-40 seconds or until smooth. Add more soy milk if you like a smoothie of thinner consistency.
3. Pour into tall glasses and serve with crushed ice.

Cottage Cheese and Spiced Raspberry Smoothie

Serves: 1

Ingredients:

- ¼ cup cottage cheese, (fat free)
- ¾ cup fresh raspberries
- 1 date
- ½ teaspoon honey
- 1 tablespoon rolled oats
- A dash ground cinnamon
- Ice cubes as required

Method:

1. Deseed the date and add into a blender. Also add raspberry, honey, cottage cheese, rolled oats and cinnamon.
2. Blend for 30-40 seconds or until smooth. Add a little water if you like a smoothie of thinner consistency.
3. Pour into tall glasses and serve.

BLUEBERRY CHEESECAKE SMOOTHIE

Serves: 1

Ingredients:

- ½ cup frozen blueberries
- 14 cup cold water
- ¼ teaspoon vanilla extract
- ½ cup skim milk
- ¼ cup low fat cottage cheese
- 2 teaspoons Splenda or Stevia drops to taste
- ¼ teaspoon ground cinnamon

Method:

1. Add blueberries, skim milk, cold water, cottage cheese, cinnamon, Stevia and vanilla into a blender. Blend for 30-40 seconds or until smooth. Add more skim milk if you like a smoothie of thinner consistency.
2. Pour into tall glasses and serve with crushed ice.

GINGERY STRAWBERRY AND KALE SMOOTHIE

Serves: 1

Ingredients:

- 3 large fresh curly kale leaves
- ¾ cup fresh strawberries
- ¼ cup cold water
- 1 inch piece fresh ginger
- 1 ½ tablespoons lime juice
- 1 teaspoon honey
- Ice cubes as required

Method:

1. Hull and chop the strawberries. Tear the kale leaves.
2. Peel the ginger and grate it.
3. Add strawberries, kale, cold water, ginger, lime juice, honey and ice cubes into a blender.
4. Blend for 30-40 seconds or until smooth. Add more water if you want a smoothie of thinner consistency.
5. Pour into a tall glass and serve.

<u>Red Currant and Pear Smoothie</u>

Serves: 2

Ingredients:

- 1 cup red currants
- 1 medium pear
- 1 cup soy milk

Method:

1. Peel, core and chop the pear. You can leave the peel intact for more nutrients.
2. Add all the ingredients into a blender.
3. Blend for 30-40 seconds or until smooth. Add more soy milk if you like a smoothie of thinner consistency.
4. Pour into tall glasses and serve with crushed ice.

BERRY AND SPINACH SMOOTHIE

Serves: 2

Ingredients:

- 1 cup almond milk, unsweetened
- 1 cup Greek yogurt
- 1 cup spinach
- 1 cup baby kale
- 2 oranges
- 1 cup mixed berries of your choice, frozen

Method:

1. Peel and deseed the oranges. Chop into pieces.
2. Add almond milk, oranges, yogurt, spinach, kale, and berries into a blender.
3. Blend for 30-40 seconds or until smooth. Add more almond milk if you like a smoothie of thinner consistency.
4. Pour into tall glasses and serve with crushed ice.

Don't forget to like this book and leave a review!

LEAN AND GREEN SMOOTHIE

Serves: 2

Ingredients:

- 5 cups kale leaves
- 1 ½ cups fresh apple juice, chilled
- 1 Granny Smith apple
- 1 cup green grapes, seedless, frozen
- A few fresh green grapes, halved to garnish
- 2 cups pineapple chunks
- Ice cubes as required

Method:

1. Add kale, apple juice, apple, frozen green grapes, pineapple chunks and ice cubes into a blender.
2. Blend for 30-40 seconds or until smooth.
3. Pour into tall glasses. Garnish with halved grapes and serve.

SUNRISE SMOOTHIE

Serves: 1

Ingredients:

- ¾ cup water melon cubes
- 2 tablespoons orange juice
- ½ cup cantaloupe cubes
- ¼ cup low fat plain yogurt
- Small wedges of cantaloupe or water melon to serve

Method:

1. Deseed the water melon and cantaloupe pieces.
2. Add watermelon cubes into the blender.
3. Blend for 30-40 seconds or until smooth.
4. Pour into a tall glass.
5. Clean the blender. Add cantaloupe, orange juice and yogurt into the blender.
6. Carefully pour the cantaloupe puree over the water melon in the glass. Do not stir.
7. Garnish with cantaloupe or water melon and serve immediately.

Carrot Smoothie

Serves: 2

Ingredients:

- 4 medium carrots
- 2 cups orange juice
- 1 teaspoon orange zest
- Ice cubes as required
- Orange peel curls to serve

Method:

1. Peel and slice the carrots.
2. Place a saucepan over medium heat. Add water and bring to the boil.
3. Add carrots.
4. Lower heat and cover the saucepan with a lid. Simmer until the carrots are soft.
5. Drain and cool the carrots completely.
6. Add carrots, orange zest, orange juice and ice cubes into a blender.
7. Blend for 30-40 seconds or until smooth.
8. Pour into tall glasses. Garnish with orange peel curls and serve right away.

Super Berry Smoothie

Serves: 2

Ingredients:

- 1 cup strawberries
- ½ cup blackberries or blueberries
- ½ cup raspberries
- ½ cup pomegranate juice
- ½ cup fresh spinach leaves
- 1 ½ tablespoons diabetic friendly vanilla protein powder

Method:

1. Rinse and tear the spinach leaves.
2. Add spinach, pomegranate juice, protein powder and berries into a blender.
3. Blend for 30-40 seconds or until smooth. Add more pomegranate juice if you like a smoothie of thinner consistency.
4. Pour into tall glasses and serve with crushed ice.

Blueberry and Almond Smoothie

Serves: 1

Ingredients:

- ¾ cup fresh blueberries
- 2 tablespoons almonds, chopped
- 2 tablespoons almond milk, unsweetened
- ¼ cup plain fat free Greek yogurt
- 1 tablespoons wheat germ
- 1 teaspoon honey

Method:

1. Add blueberries, almonds, almond milk, yogurt, wheat germ and honey into a blender.
2. Blend for 30-40 seconds or until smooth.
3. Pour into a tall glass and serve with crushed ice.

PEANUT BUTTER RASPBERRY SMOOTHIE

Serves: 1

Ingredients:

- ¾ cup fresh raspberries
- 1 tablespoon natural smooth peanut butter
- 1 tablespoon skim milk
- 1 teaspoon honey
- ½ cup ice cubes

Method:

1. Add raspberries, peanut butter, skim milk, honey and ice cubes into a blender.
2. Blend for 30-40 seconds or until smooth.
3. Pour into a tall glass and serve.

APPLE SPINACH SMOOTHIE

Serves: 1

Ingredients:

- ½ small apple
- ¼ cup plain fat free Greek yogurt
- 1 tablespoon ground flaxseeds
- 1 cup packed baby spinach
- 3 tablespoons fresh apple juice or orange juice
- ½ teaspoon maple syrup
- Ice cubes as required

Method:

1. Core and chop the apple.
2. Add apple, spinach, yogurt, apple juice, ground flaxseeds, maple syrup and ice into a blender.
3. Blend for 30-40 seconds or until smooth.
4. Pour into a tall glass and serve.

NUTTY BLACKBERRY SMOOTHIE

Serves: 1

Ingredients:

- ¾ cup fresh blackberries
- 1 tablespoon almond butter
- ¼ cup plain fat free Greek yogurt
- 1 teaspoon honey
- Ice cubes as required
-

Method:

1. Add blackberries, almond butter, yogurt, honey and ice cubes into a blender.
2. Blend for 30-40 seconds or until smooth.
3. Pour into a tall glass and serve.

BLUEBERRY PINEAPPLE AND COCONUT SMOOTHIE

Serves: 3

Ingredients:

- 1 cup blueberries
- 1 cup pineapple pieces
- 1 cup coconut water or coconut milk
- 1 inch piece fresh ginger

Method:

1. Peel the ginger and grate it.
2. Add blueberries, pineapple pieces, coconut milk or coconut water and ginger into a blender.
3. Blend for 30-40 seconds or until smooth. Add more coconut water or coconut milk if you want a smoothie of thinner consistency.
4. Pour into tall glasses and serve with crushed ice.

BERRY SMOOTHIE BOWL

Serves: 1

Ingredients:

- ¾ cup plain low-fat Greek yogurt
- ½ tablespoon almond butter
- ½ tablespoon chia seeds
- ½ teaspoon coconut flakes, unsweetened, to garnish
- ¾ cup frozen mixed berries of your choice
- ½ tablespoon hemp hearts
- 2 tablespoons coconut water or water
- Fresh berries to garnish

Method:

1. Add yogurt, almond butter, chia seeds, berries, hemp hearts and coconut water into a blender.
2. Blend for 30-40 seconds or until smooth.
3. Pour into a bowl. Garnish with fresh berries and coconut flakes.
4. Serve right away or chill and serve later.

Low Sugar Green Smoothie Bowl

Serves: 1

Ingredients:

- ½ cup coconut milk or coconut milk or unsweetened almond milk
- ½ cup spinach
- 1 ½ cups assorted kale like curly and lacinato etc.
- ½ ripe avocado
- ½ small banana, frozen
- 1 Brazil nut
- ½ teaspoon ground cinnamon
- ¼ teaspoon ground ginger
- ½ date, pitted
- 1 teaspoon moringa powder
- A pinch salt
- ½ scoop protein powder or collagen powder
- 2 teaspoons almond butter
- ½ teaspoon turmeric powder
- Ice cubes as required
- Kiwi slices to serve
- 1 teaspoon chia seeds to serve
- 1 teaspoon coconut flakes, unsweetened to serve

Method:

1. Discard hard ribs and stem of the kale. Tear the kale leaves.
2. Add all the ingredients except kiwi, chia seeds and coconut flakes into a blender.
3. Blend for 30-40 seconds or until smooth.

4. Pour into a bowl. Sprinkle chia seeds and coconut flakes. Garnish with kiwi slices and serve.

Don't forget to like this book and leave a review!

Conclusion

Who doesn't like a glass of good smoothie that is full of flavor and nutrients? Not only are smoothies healthy, they are extremely easy to make and hassle free!

If you want to create a perfect glass of creamy smoothie, then you will need to be mindful of the timing, amount of water added to it, and the kitchen appliance you are using. Here are a few tips that you can keep in mind while making a smoothie. A smoothie needs some refrigeration time for attaining that perfect creamy consistency. The ingredients in it will soak up all the water when the ice cubes melt and provide the creamy texture. For obtaining that gooey and thick consistency, add some chia seeds or flax seeds. If the smoothie ends up getting too thick, then add a little bit of water or coconut milk can help in diluting it.

Make sure that you steer clear of canned fruits since they have hidden sugars in them. Make use of seasonal fruits and if that's not possible, you can opt for frozen fruits. Do not add sugar to your smoothies. Instead, you can make use of natural sweeteners like some raw honey or Stevia. You will need to stock up your pantry with the necessary ingredients and that's about it. These recipes don't require any fancy ingredients and everything you need can be acquired from the local supermarket. The next time you feel like having some dessert, you can whip up a smoothie instead. You can satiate your craving for something sweet without having to worry about all the calories and sugar. Isn't that wonderful?

The recipes that have been mentioned in this book are diabetic friendly. Also, one glass of power packed smoothie can help you in obtaining more than half of your daily nutritional needs. This healthy drink is easy to make and the prep isn't time-consuming. Make the most of your power blender and start making these nutritionally rich smoothies. You don't have to be an expert for whipping up this glass of goodness. Once you get a hang of the flavor combinations that work together, you can start experimenting with different ingredients! Depending on your personal taste, you can tweak these recipes as well. So, all that is left for you to do would be to get started!

I would like to thank you once again for purchasing this book. I hope you enjoy reading this book as much as I enjoyed writing it. Don't forget to like this book and leave a review!

Thank you and all the best!

<u>Check Out My Other Books</u>

Below you'll find another one of my popular books that. Simply search for the title on the Amazon website or click on the title!

DASH Diet Made Easy: 25 DASH Diet Recipes for Beginners!

Care Less, Live More: How to Stop Giving a You Know What

www.ingramcontent.com/pod-product-compliance
Lightning Source LLC
Chambersburg PA
CBHW070055260726
48658CB00002B/881